Get  ious

Get Slim

Get ready to take back control
of your life

Barry Collins & Marina Collins

Get Serious Get Slim

Get ready to take back control of your life

Barry Collins

Marina Collins

ISBN 978-1541232761

1st Edition 2017

Foreward

If you choose to follow the recommendations in this book relating to lifestyle, diet and exercise, we recommend you ensure your medical practitioner understands and approves the changes you intend to make, *before* undertaking and dietary modifications, or physical exertion.

Whilst the guidance given in this book is suitable for the vast majority of individuals, it may not be suitable for you , due to your current health status. Please seek the advice of a medical practitioner and/or nutritionist to ensure the changes you are about to undertake will have a positive effect on your health.

Introduction

Where Do I Start?

So you've decided it's time to take back control of your health, eating and weight? I'm glad, because nothing saddens me as much as seeing someone suffer needlessly, believing that things are beyond their control. If you believed you were a victim of circumstances, or that it was because the dog stole your beans when you were 4, or that you were born with a genetic predisposition to require chocolate as much as oxygen, then I have some sad news for you... it's simply not true.

You may have wanted to believe those things, or have been told them so often and convincingly that, "It must be true," but the harsh reality is this — *you're in control...* or you will be soon!

It doesn't matter who you are, what shape or size you are, or what has prompted you to buy this book now, because that fact that you've opened it to the first page tells me one thing... you want change. I'm sure there will be people who are starting this journey at all different levels of health, fitness and diet, but that doesn't matter because you are all heading in the same direction together... towards a healthier, happier you!

Chapter 1

It's Not Your Fault
It's Not Just About Food

And therein lies the conundrum... to be healthy *and* happy. If your head is still spinning from your last ride on the diet roller coaster, you'll be all too familiar with the initial thrust of enthusiasm that comes with all that is promised if you only eat more of this, less of that and cut some stuff out altogether. but then as you settled in to the daily ups and downs of the life of a dieter, you would reward yourself when you had a good day or week, and console yourself when it all went horribly wrong. So as your health was temporarily improving your happiness was taking a nosedive as you craved all the 'forbidden' foods.

Eventually, you may have decided you were only dieting to achieve happiness, and that clearly wasn't working, so perhaps sending the diet packing and reaching for the crisps or ice cream would deliver you to your own version of heaven? Perhaps for a short time, until your initial health concerns returned, along with all the guilt associated with not taking good enough care of yourself, and you were able to climb aboard the dieters roller coaster once more.

So let me be very clear on one thing... This is *not* a diet! I'm happy to say that I can give you guidance about the foods that will help or hinder your success, however where the true changes will occur, will not be in *what* you eat, but rather in *how* you eat. My expertise lies in understanding how your thoughts translate in to your actions, and helping you to understand, so you can begin to take actions that will result in you becoming healthier and happier through thinking and feeling differently.

There's No Magic Wand

So if you've already had a flick through looking for "the secret," the revolutionary technique that will magically make you the shape and size you want, then you may be feeling slightly disappointed, but all is not lost.

When I see clients privately, one of the things they all have in common is they all tell me a version of, "I know what I should be doing...". What they don't get, at least at the start, is that they have no idea just how true that is.

If you've ever been around small children, and I mean really small, you may have noticed how, normally, they don't suffer from weight problems, certainly not like the 64% of UK adults or 70% of American adults who have a BMI (body mass index) over 25, meaning they are classed as, at best, overweight, and at worst morbidly obese. This isn't because they've already read this, or some other book, or adopted the latest health kick craze that's sweeping the nation. It's because mother nature is pretty good at her job, and can produce the almost perfect engine every time. So what happens to this near-perfect system that only consumes the fuel it needs, at the rate it needs it? Well, to be quite blunt, Life!

Think about it like this, babies don't have relationship problems, or financial burdens. They don't have self doubt and confidence issues, anxiety and stress are foreign to them, and so they only consume as much as they need, when they need it, and then they stop. If you've ever tried to give a baby the last ounce of milk or the last spoonful of food, when it's internal system says, 'no more' you'll know what I'm talking about! It's the perfect system... and then life happens!

Food no longer is just a source of energy, it becomes a friend, an enemy, a comfort and much, much more, and all this begins to happen very early. So if your relationship with food is not ideal, it's no great surprise, so stop giving yourself a hard time about it! You've spent years being reprogrammed to change mother natures programming, but the good news is, it can be reversed. So the secret contained within these pages is not a technique or juice or pill, it's this...

You already know what to do to be healthy.

Back To Basics

Because there's been so many layers, beliefs or programs, added over the years, you need to strip them away to get back to the way that works, so that's what you're going to do. You're going to reset back to being healthy! That may sound incredibly simple, and it is! If a baby only days or weeks old can do it easily, I'm confident you can too!

In the pages ahead I'll explain to you how to strip away the programs that no longer work, so that the ones that work, the ones already inside of you, can come to the surface again, and then we'll set about optimising them to make your return to health almost effortless.

Over the years there's probably been a lot of influences that have ultimately led you to become the person you are today. Some will have been well intentioned, and some not so. What's important as you begin to change is you become aware of *how* you've been influenced over the years so that you can stop any negative influences in their tracks and immerse yourself in the good stuff, the stuff that will continually move you closer to your goals.

Babies & Blue Minis

I don't know if you've ever had the experience of buying a car from a garage. You go along and you might spend a few hours eliminating ones that aren't suitable, you test drive a few, you might even sleep on it before you eventually settle on a blue Mini (other car manufacturers are available) and agree a collection date a week or so later, during which time your thoughts are dominated by your soon to be new car...

And then a peculiar thing begins to happen. You begin to notice things around you have changed. The guy at the end of the road drives the same car as your new one, so does the woman opposite you at the traffic lights, and the family next to you in the car park... before you know it you're seeing blue Minis everywhere!

I had a similar conversation with a client, and she told me how she had just recently taken ownership of a silver BMW, and had experienced exactly what I have described. For the next couple of days, I can't tell you how many silver BMWs I saw, but it was a lot. This simply shows that the programming of your unconscious to focus on something isn't complicated, or difficult, in fact it's so easy it can happen by accident, unless you make a choice to use it to your advantage.

If you or your partner has ever been pregnant, and your thoughts are filled with all the things you need to buy, buggies, prams, cots, blankets, bottles, nappies. You might consider your health more, taking vitamins, planning maternity leave...

Suddenly you become aware the woman in the next office has just gone off on maternity leave, and it seems like everybody at the supermarket has a baby in the trolley, your friends are all talking about starting a families and how their friends are all having babies too.

Now, the world has not really changed in response to your impending arrival (car or baby), but your window of awareness has been opened, and you are now *consciously* acknowledging these things which have always been there, invisible, but still seeping in to your unconscious.

Now think back to every time you were told, "If you eat any more pizza, you'll turn in to a pizza," or "You can't have that, it's fattening" and "Your just big like the rest of the family," and slowly your attention becomes filled with all the ways you can gain weight, and the ways you can move steadily towards poor health and unhappiness.

What I'm highlighting is this...

What you focus on, you get more of!

So whilst initially it might seem like a good idea to have your 'fat' photo on the refrigerator door to serve as a warning reminder of what you're fighting against, it's simply focusing your attention in the completely wrong direction, and where the mind leads, the body will follow. People who suffer from weight problems commonly accept their current situation as part of their identity. By this, I mean people who are overweight will frequently consider themselves 'fat' while those who are underweight view themselves as skinny. They are not, they are simply engaging in behaviours that will most likely result in one particular body shape or another. If you changed career path, and gave up being a goat herder to become a ballet dancer, you would no longer be a goat herder. You would understand the experience of herding goats, but having decided it's no longer what you want to do, you have adopted a new set of behaviours (dancing), but that still wouldn't mean it's your identity... you would no more be a dancer than you were a goat herder. You are just you - dancing (or herding goats) is what you do, not who you are. Become aware of what you are focusing on, and make a choice about how you view yourself.

You are not a goat herder or a dancer, and you are *certainly not a weight!* Some people get fixated on the number they see on the scales, becoming obsessed with the natural rise and fall that *everyone* experiences, even when they're not aware of it. So if you absolutely *must* see a number changing (getting bigger *or* smaller), I'll give you a way to achieve this later on...

What I would much rather you do is this: Get a photo of yourself when you were really happy with the way you looked, when you felt really confident and comfortable in your body, and put that on the refrigerator door. If you don't have a picture of yourself, find one that represents the ideal you. Do you have a dress or suit hiding at the back of the wardrobe, the "maybe one day" outfit? Then get it out, and hang it at the front of your wardrobe or on the mirror, somewhere where you will see it, at the very least, daily, but preferably more than once per day! This will begin to focus your attention on where you're going, not where you've been.

As you make your way through this book, and begin to make positive changes in your life, you will become aware of the behaviours that have become second nature to you and have led to your unhealthy lifestyle. Firstly, feel good that you have identified them now rather than later, and secondly, make the decision to resolve these issues before they take you any further down the route you were previously on. I know you might be tempted to look back at everything you've done and give yourself a hard time for all the things you will become aware of, but let me ask you this... will it make you feel good, and will it change the past? If the answer is no (and I suspect it is) then don't do it, just be grateful you have the opportunity now to make changes before it becomes too late. Remember, you can't change something you don't know you're doing, so becoming aware of these behaviours is the positive first step to lasting change.

So before you go any further, I'd like you to write down 3 things that you want to achieve framed in the positive. When I ask this question, I'll frequently get a list of things my clients don't want e.g. I don't want to be the size I am; I don't want to buy big, baggy clothes anymore; I wish I didn't feel so horrible when I look in the mirror. From now on I want you to focus on what you do want e.g. I want to be 3 sizes smaller; I want to be able to run in the park with my children; I want to be able to buy fashionable clothes. Remember, what you focus on, you get more of, so, what do you want?

1.

2.

3.

Chapter 2

Exercise
Slow & steady wins the race

Treadmill Trepidation

So when does the change begin? It will begin as soon as you decide to make it happen, because it doesn't happen by itself. You need to be an active participant in the process. Imagine if you had a personal trainer at the gym, and 5 days a week, you go to the gym and watch your trainer doing a workout, showing you which exercises work this group of muscles, which exercises will tone that group of muscles, and then you go home and slob on the sofa. Who is going to reap the benefits of those workouts, you or your trainer?

This is the bit where I mention the 'E' word... EXERCISE! But before you throw this book away in disgust, take a moment and just notice the rate of your breathing. Now, if you can, notice your pulse. Now think about all the things you probably do every day that cause you to breath harder than you're doing right now, and make your pulse beat faster than it is just now. I'm not talking about doing an hour on the treadmill, getting hot and sweaty. I'm talking about being more active by doing the things you can do comfortably.

Now obviously as with any course of physical activity, discuss with your medical practitioner to ensure that any activity you are about to undertake is going to have a positive effect and is within your ability. The sort of thing I'm suggesting to begin with is getting off the bus one stop early on the way home from work, parking at the far end of the car park when you go to the supermarket, take the dog for an extra lap of the park. I suppose I should really call it extra activity instead of exercise, because it's things you're already doing daily and just deciding to do a little bit more of them. Now I know it may not seem like a lot when you start out but stick with it and you'll soon begin to feel the benefits and you'll notice that you'll be more comfortable afterwards, as your breathing is less laboured and your pulse is racing less.

One Step At A Time

Where you're aiming for is being able to do some form of activity for 10 minutes per day. When you can do that for 3 consecutive days, increase the time by 2 minutes. Once you can comfortably do 12 minutes per day for 3 consecutive days, increase it to 14 minutes, and so on...

If you can't manage 10 minutes per day to begin with, then find the time you can do, and start from there.

Another approach is to monitor your steps using a pedometer, either a stand alone one, although many smartphones have them built in now. Over a few days monitor how many steps you're taking, and you'll get an idea what your personal average is. Once you know that, aim to increase it by 25% over the next two weeks. For example, if your average number of steps per day is 6000, then in two weeks time aim to have that daily average hitting 8000 steps.

So now that the thought of extra activity is not so scary, here's the good news... You get to feel good for no reason at all!

When you exercise you body releases chemicals called endorphins, natures feel good drugs, that flood your system, and actively lift your mood. They also have the benefit of being a natural analgesic, or pain reliever, so you can always start any activity knowing you're going to feel even better afterwards.

Although there is no 'chemical' addiction to what is sometimes called the "runners high," there's nothing wrong with understanding what makes you happy and healthy at the same time and realising, you want to do more!

Finding The Balance

You can make this process as simple, or as complicated as you want, but I much prefer to keep things simple, because if it were too complicated, people would get overwhelmed, and go back to what they know, even though they know what they were doing didn't work.

So with that in mind, here's why activity is an integral part of your new lifestyle.

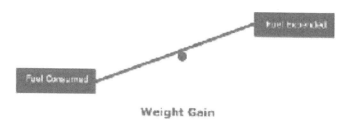

Weight Gain

If you are consuming food (fuel) at a level that is in excess of the demands of your body (the engine), the result is weight gain and all that extra fuel is going to have to be stored somewhere, and *you're* the one thats going to have to carry it around with you everywhere you go.

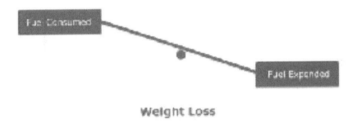

Weight Loss

If your fuel intake (food) is slightly lower than the consumption (energy used during activity), then as well as using the fuel you've just taken on board, you'll use a little of the reserves you had built up too, resulting in weight loss.

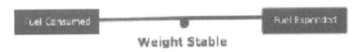

Weight Stable

Once you've achieved a healthy weight and are healthy & happy, matching the fuel and the consumption levels, results in a stable weight, allowing you to maintain your healthy lifestyle.

So depending on where you are at right now, will determine the route to follow to achieve you desired outcome.

Use the space below write down 3 things you already do, that you can do for 10 minutes a day and will enjoy doing more of.

1.

2.

3.

Use this space to record your progress in either steps or time as described earlier in the chapter.

Day 1 - Steps / time:	Day 7 - Steps / time:
Day 14 - Steps / time:	Day 21 - Steps / time:
Day 28 - Steps / time:	Day 35 - Steps / time:

Chapter 3

Hunger Scale
Hitting The Reset Button

Stop The Ride, I Want To Get Off

If you've done the whole diet rollercoaster in the past, you've been teaching you body to override it's natural ability to regulate fuel, and successfully managed to put your metabolism in feast or famine mode.

This goes all the way back to caveman days when, if food is plentiful (feast), your body recognises that it's getting more fuel than is needed, so begins to store extra in preparation for scarcity. When 'famine' comes, and food is less readily available, your body tries to conserve energy and fuel, by slowing your metabolism down, and burning as little of the fuel reserves as possible. Fortunately, your reality is probably very different to that and it's quite likely you have access to plentiful supply of nutrition pretty much all the time, right?

So either your day was planned around opening and closing times of cafes & restaurants, and your route home takes you past the widest possible range of take aways to ensure you're never left wanting. Getting home, you might grab a bottle of something fizzy as you head for the sofa for a little 'me' time with your takeaway, before spending the remainder of the evening rubbing your fit-to-burst stomach as you gently chastise yourself for having overdone it.

Or you might be working with the "if-I-eat-less-I'll-weigh-less" approach... You have the first of many coffees for breakfast, lunch happens on the third Thursday of the month when you have to go to head office for a meeting, but you're a trooper and your caffeine intake powers you through the day. Dinner is a rice cake, generously lathered in the lowest low-fat spread you can find, as you dream of something as full of flavour as polystyrene or cardboard, before almost fainting in to bed, wondering why you just can't get rid of this headache!

Ok, so both these examples are a bit extreme, but there may still be parts of it that you recognise in yourself. I wouldn't be surprised if you did.

Good news time again... you're not going to need to learn something new, in fact I'm going to ask you to forget many of the 'rules' you believed were going to help you get back in control, and begin the process of resetting.

Some people tell me, "I'm never hungry" whilst others tell me, "I'm always hungry". Now obviously, neither of these statements can be completely true, however that doesn't mean it's not how that person perceives their satiety, or hunger levels.

Please Sir, Can I Have Some More?

If you are of a certain age (ahem), then as a child you probably heard all about the starving children in Africa, most probably as you sat at the dinner table trying to strike a bargain so you wouldn't need to finish whatever it was that remained on your plate, all the time considering whether or not your parents would indeed give you half a kipper with steamed cabbage for tomorrows breakfast if you didn't finish it.

I had a client who explained to me that as a child during the war, she came from a 'wealthy' family. That meant a family who could give their children fresh fruit! In her class at primary school there were twins who would follow her around at break times in the hope that when she finished her apple, she would give them the core to share between them because that was the only fresh fruit they get. And so you can understand that a family that could scrape together enough money to put good food on the table, would not want to see it going to waste. I'm sure you get that, but what's not the same is the world we live in. What is still the same is when you're full, you're full!

Yes, your stomach can accommodate more food than it takes to make you feel full, but we're not living in a famine, so you can comfortably stop when you feel satisfied without having to eat to the point where it used to hurt. Most people are surprised to discover that the volume of food it takes to satisfy you is roughly the same size as your clenched fist.

Before you go any further, answer this... are you hungry right now?

What was your answer, yes, no? Sorry, but it's a trick question. Your satiety level is not an either-or sensation, there are a range of sensations and experiences.

1. Physically Faint

2. Ravenous

3. **Fairly hungry**

4. **Slightly hungry**

5. **<u>Neutral</u>**

6. **Pleasantly satisfied**

7. **Full**

8. Stuffed

9. Bloated

10. Nauseous

The Hunger Scale

You may have had the experience of being so hungry that it physically affects you, light headedness, hands shaking, lack of concentration... This would be classed as *physically faint*.

The sensation of cramping in the stomach, causing discomfort would be *ravenous*.

The sensation in your stomach that lets you know its about to rumble would put you firmly in the *fairly hungry* category, it's the 'I need to stop what I'm doing and eat now' feeling

Slightly hungry is characterised in that moment when you realise you're beginning to get a bit peckish, and know you're going to need something to eat within the next 90 minutes or so.

If you find you are neither hungry or satisfied, you're probably *neutral*.

When you finish eating and feel sated, but know you could comfortably eat a little more if it were offered, would indicate you're *pleasantly satisfied*.

When you notice that the food has lost some of its appeal, or you might feel a sensation like a weight settling at the top of your stomach, just below your rib cage, this would suggest you are *full*.

After eating, if you feel the need to take out the button on your trousers, to let your dinner settle, and perhaps feel a bit sluggish, then you're probably *stuffed*.

If you reach the point of pain just below your rib cage, or along the collar bone, then you have achieved *bloated*.

When you feel a lump at the base of your throat, find it difficult to swallow, sometimes accompanied by a fine sheen of sweat on your face, then you're probably *nauseous*.

So now that you have a better understanding of your personal experience of satiety or hunger, I'll ask that questions again in a slightly different way. On the hunger scale from one to ten, where would you place yourself right now? Take a moment to consider your answer. Close your eyes and 'check in' with yourself. Look beyond whats going on in your head, to become aware of the sensations in your stomach, and answer the question based on this.

Now consider when you last ate, and how much you had to eat, and figure in how active you've been since you ate as well. Do all of these factors match your experience? If you had a light meal 4 or 5 hours ago, but have been out working in the garden, I'd expect you to feel *fairly* or *slightly hungry*. If you had a large meal within the last couple of hours and have been sitting with a good book (this one perhaps?) since then, I'd expect you to feel *pleasantly satisfied* or *full*. Now this may not match your experience exactly, but I'm sure you get the idea. If the sensations you are experiencing don't quite tally with what you have eaten and your activity levels, then this simply demonstrates what we already know, you're awareness of you hunger levels is in need of recalibration.

The important thing is that you check in with how you feel physically, and not how you feel emotionally! You may not get it right every time to begin with, and that's all right, as you begin to recalibrate your awareness of hunger and satiety, you'll get better at it. How? You calibrate regularly, every hour, in fact. Every hour, while you're awake, take a moment to check in with your hunger levels and begin to notice the small distinctions between one level and the next. It's not a big job, it is just taking 20 or 30 seconds to turn your attention inwards and assess how hungry you feel physically. I would expect you to be doing this hourly for at least the first few weeks, to help your body recalibrate your awareness easily.

What you will begin to notice is that throughout the day your hunger levels will drop gradually and inline with your activity levels - If you're doing something more active you will move from *full* to *fairly hungry* quicker than if you are using less energy.

Emotional Hunger

Watch out for sudden changes in your hunger levels. This can be an indication of emotional hunger.

In the past, you may have experienced emotional hunger, which can be identified by the way it suddenly comes on. By checking in regularly with your hunger level, you'll notice when you move from seven to six, to five, and suddenly to a two, sometimes after an event, or thought, that causes a change in your emotional state. The other clue is when you notice that what you want is a specific food to satisfy your desire.

Genuine hunger can be sated with any food. Cravings, boredom and emotional eating can all be characterised by their need for a specific taste e.g. "I want chocolate". If you're uncertain if it is a craving or genuine hunger, apply a little common sense. When was the last time you ate, and how much energy have you used since then? Hunger also works in approximately 90 minute cycles, although the vast majority of people find this doubles (roughly) to a three to four hour cycle, so consider this when thinking about how long since you last ate. Have a glass of water, as dehydration can also sometimes manifest itself as a hunger that can't quite be satisfied, but we'll look at this in more detail later.

What I would recommend is using a 'food diary' like the one at the end of this chapter to record when and what you're eating, but also noting where your hunger level was before *and* after you ate. Write the day in the left hand column, and your food & drink in the larger boxes to the right. In the two smaller boxes above, note down your hunger levels before and afterwards.

This will help you to identify any unwanted patterns that are holding you back, and also the one that will promote good health. You'll also notice patterns of food that you repeatedly have and how that is affecting your progress.

On the far right you can also record what 'extra activity' you've done (see chapter 3).

Breakfast	Snack	Lunch	Snack	Dinner	Snack	Exercise

	Day one	Day Two	Day Three

Chapter 4

Eat When You Are Hungry
Metabolic tune up

So let me ask you that question a slightly different way, how hungry are you right now? Rate your hunger levels using the descriptions in the previous chapter, and notice how hungry you really feel, not how hungry you think you should be. If you've just had something to eat I'd expect you feel somewhere from 5 to 10, if it's a while since you've eaten you may be between 1 and 5.

The process of bringing your body out of fat storing mode (feast or famine, remember), is done by maintaining your hunger-satiety levels between levels 3 to 7. By making sure you are always 3 or higher, and 7 or below, teaches your body that fuel (food) is not in short supply, nor is it likely to be anytime soon. Your body will soon learn that there is no need store and conserve fat by slowing your metabolism down. As your body learns that fuel is supplied when it is needed (you eat when you're hungry) and that you are not preparing for famine (you stop when you feel full), you will begin to let go of the fat stores you were holding on to - in other words, you will lose weight.

If we think about babies and how they deal with hunger, they are very aware of the sensation of being hungry, and most will let you know quite loudly if that need is not met. When you're performing your hourly checks notice when you get to 4, and consider what you're doing over the next hour or so. If you're about to go in to a 3 hour meeting at work, it would be wise to have a snack now to ensure you don't drop below 3.

On the other hand if your next meal is only 20 minutes away, and feel confident you won't drop below 3 in that time, then head for dinner table. In other words, become aware of becoming more hungry and use your best judgement, but make sure...

When you are hungry, EAT!

Giving your body the fuel it needs, when it needs it, teaches your body that it doesn't need the reserves of fuel it's been creating until now. Over time, as you continue to supply the right amount of fuel, at the right time, and your body begins to relinquish the reserves it's been holding on to, and gently, steadily you will begin to notice your clothes, where once tight and uncomfortable, will begin to become more comfortable and loose fitting.

You had most likely been systematically programmed throughout your life to override and ignore the signals that your body sends you to let you know it needs more fuel. Genuine hunger, and by that I mean a need for food, comes on gradually, so by checking in hourly with your hunger levels you will begin to notice the small distinctions in the sensation as you move from six to five, to four, and eventually to three.

I don't know if you've ever noticed that when you have breakfast, ideally within an hour of waking, that within a few hours you find you are hungry again? Conversely, if you skip breakfast, you can last 5 or 6 hours without really feeling hungry. You were probably told as a child that breakfast is the most important meal of the day, but never really questioned why. Let me explain...

When you skip breakfast, but then start going about your daily routine, which will involve you using energy, your body identifies that it's using energy that it hasn't had the proper supplies for because you skipped breakfast. To compensate, your body reduces your metabolic rate to conserve the fuel reserves it has, effectively reducing the rate at which you burn fat, making it even harder to lose weight.

However, when you *do* have breakfast, your body recognises that fuel is being supplied to provide for the activity taking place, and as long as you continue this trend, your body learns that fuel is plentiful and can use as much as it needs, and has no need for the fuel reserves you had been laboriously carrying in the form of fat, and so begins to gently deplete these reserves, which results in weight loss. As your metabolic rate accelerates, burning through more fuel, you will become aware of the feeling of hunger more frequently.

Think of your metabolism like a steam engine. If it's just ticking along gently, you'll only need to fuel the furnace infrequently. If you increase your speed, you'll find the furnace goes through more fuel, and you'll need to tend to it more frequently, if you don't keep refuelling, then the fire will go out, and you will need to start from the beginning again to build up the fire!

The secret to your success is in learning how much is the right amount of fuel to take on - too little and you're heading back in to famine. Too much and you'll suffocate the furnace and begin to lose momentum. If you've ever had a meal so heavy that afterwards, all you want to do is have a nap, you know exactly what this feel like!

Chapter 5

Stop when you are full

"So how do I know when I've had the right amount?" I hear you ask...

Think about the hungry babies again for a moment, and remember the example I gave of trying to get them to take one more mouthful. My experience is that you're more likely to end up wearing it or decorating the walls with it, than it getting eaten!

As you continue to recalibrate your awareness through hourly checks of your hunger levels, pay particular attention to when you're eating. Start by calibrating just before you start to eat, and continue to check between mouthfuls, until you become aware of the small moves up the scale as you move from *fairly hungry* to *full*. When you reach 6, you'll learn that the feeling of being *full* is not far away, and then...

When you are full, STOP!

Now that might seem like common sense, but it's not as common as it should be. So many people spent their childhoods being conditioned to eat when they were full or not hungry, or not eating when they were actually hungry, so whilst it does make sense, it's not that common for people to be actually living this way!

Have you ever gone to the supermarket on an empty stomach? How much extra food did you buy on impulse, because you could imagine it satisfying your hunger right there and then. This is what people commonly do at mealtimes, they fill out their portions based on how they feel at the beginning of the meal. If you've allowed yourself to get to 'fairly hungry', then you were probably inclined to fill out more than you will actually need, or enjoy! As a result you would possibly have overeaten, missing the signals that your body sends to let you know you are full.

The problem this creates is this... what does your body do with all the extra fuel? It stores it, of course. And how do you think it's stored? In fat cells! So it's not just about what foods you eat, although that plays a part too, but how you eat plays an equally important part in managing your weight.

Your body is designed to take in as much fuel as it's using, so by consistently over-fuelling your body has to make adjustments to accommodate this. It does this by muting the signals that your body sends out saying, "That's enough" so that you can consume more without being aware of how much excess you were having.

Think about your favourite meal for a moment, and remember the last time you had it. As you remember all the flavours and textures your mouth might even be watering. Now fast forward to the end of the meal and the last mouthful, and notice that whilst it was still pleasant, is was no where near as satisfying as the first. This is because when your stomach reaches capacity, a signal is sent to your brain to let it know that you are full. In response, your brain begins to reduce the amount of pleasure you get from the food by regulating dopamine production in the brain, to discourage you from continuing to eat. However having spent a large part of your childhood being reminded that, "there are starving children in Africa, and you'll be having cold stew, mushy peas and lumpy potatoes for breakfast if you don't clear your plate" you have probably become quite proficient at ignoring these signals, but they are still there - You simply need to be alert to them!

So when you sit down to a meal, before you take the first mouthful, assess just how hungry you actually are using the same scale as earlier. Here it is again...

1.   Physically faint

2.   Ravenous

3.   **Fairly hungry**

4.   **Slightly hungry**

5.   **<u>Neutral</u>**

6.   **Pleasantly satisfied**

7.   **Full**

8.   Stuffed

9.   Bloated

10. Nauseous

And as you proceed to eat your meal, check in with your satiety level between mouthfuls, noticing the change as you progress from three through to seven. Remember, when you are full, STOP! That's when you truly *feel* full, not when you *think* you're full. Let me explain...

I once saw a test where a random cafe was selected one morning, and a poll was taken recording everything the diners had for breakfast e.g. one sausage, two eggs, tea, two bits of toast, etc. What was recorded was not what they ordered, but what they actually ate.

The next day, the same people we're invited to return, and were served the same as they had eaten the day before, with one difference... they were all blindfolded. Can you guess what happened? Every single person left food on their plate, many as much as half, uneaten. How did this happen? With the external reference (how much food is still on the plate) removed, the only reference they have to check in with, is their own satiety level, or in other words, do they feel full?

Where I come from, there is an expression, "Your eyes are bigger than your belly." What it commonly means is that you're filling out more food than you'll be able to eat, however the subtext is that you are measuring how much food is required to satisfy you, by looking at the food, not by the way you feel.

So by checking in with how you feel between mouthfuls will help you recalibrate your awareness of how it *feels* to be full. To begin with you may become over zealous in your efforts to get it right, and may be uncertain about if you are indeed full, or just thinking you should be. So if you *think* you are full, STOP! Check back in with how you feel in 5 or 10 minutes, and if it turns out you were a little premature, just refer back to the previous step - Eat when you're hungry. Just remember to keep checking between mouthfuls to ensure you correctly identify when you do feel *full*.

Chapter 6
Eat Consciously
Stacking the odds in your favour

The reality for many is that we have become so disconnected from our bodies and the signals it's sending all the time, it's no great surprise that obesity is the problem it is. Much of the attitude we have to food has come from our parents, and their parents before them. That's not to say it is wrong, but is it as appropriate for the world we live in today?

Thankfully there is more 'warm, fed and dry' in the world than ever before, although still not enough in my opinion, but if you're reading this, it's probably fair for me to assume that you can count on regularly getting the meals you need day after day.

And yet individuals still believe they should make their children sit at the table till their plate is clean, which simply perpetuates the problem and the associated behaviours, and builds on the foundations of obesity already present from previous generations.

Make meal times about the meal. Do you ever go to the cinema? Do you wear a blindfold when you go? Of course not! If you've gone to the effort of arranging a babysitter, making sure you've got the money, and the means to get there, and you've taken time to choose a movie that has your favourite actor and sounds like a story you'll enjoy, why, when you get there, would you deliberately deprive yourself of a large part of the experience? It doesn't make sense, and yet this is what so many do with their food.

They choose a recipe that has all their favourite ingredients, they go to the shop to get everything they need, they take the time to prepare the meal, and then pick up a book, turn on the television or open up their laptop whilst consuming their meal. They are not focusing on their meal, and in the process are most likely going to miss the signal that says, "I'm full" when it comes.

To ensure firstly that you are aware of the 'full' signal, but also to change the way you feel about food, eat consciously. That means giving your food your full attention.

Start by getting rid of all unnecessary distractions. Turn the television off, put the book or your phone down. Is that important work email really *more* important than your health? Pull the car over and take 10 minutes to focus on, and thoroughly enjoy, your food. Take the time to become fully aware of the textures, the smells, the tastes, every nuance of your tasty snack or your full meal. Eating this way, by paying attention, changes your relationship with food to make eating a pleasurable, enjoyable experience, not something to feel ashamed of, not something you do alone, that you feel you have to hide for fear of being judged.

To make this even easier for you, there are a number of small changes you can make in your behaviour until these new healthy ways become even more natural to you.

Chew each mouthful of food at least 12 times before you swallow. I'm sure you were probably told this as a child, but you might be surprised to know why this makes a difference. The enzymes that break food down are more concentrated in your saliva than in your stomach acid, and so this helps aid digestion. You can also put your cutlery down (or your food if it's finger food) between mouthfuls, not picking it up until you have swallowed.

This has the knock on effect of slowing down the speed at which you eat, giving your brain more of an opportunity to recognise the 'full' signal sent from the stomach telling you it's time to stop.

Switch your cutlery over in your hands. If you normally hold the fork in your left hand

and knife in your right, switch them over (fork in your right hand, knife in your left) to further reduce the pace you eat, increasing the time to identify the signs of being full.

Eat from a smaller plate, or fill out half portions, and only when you have eaten what's on your place, consider whether or not you are still hungry, and at this point decide how much more you can comfortably enjoy without over eating.

By following these a simple guidelines you will be eliminating many of the unconscious behaviours that lead to weight problems. By paying attention to your hunger levels between mouthfuls as you eat consciously, you will begin to notice any remaining behaviours that are holding you back, and then begin to address these easily, as once you have conscious awareness of these problem behaviours, they are far easier to eliminate.

Chapter 7

Eat The Food You Enjoy
So what should you eat?

The next time you're in the supermarket, sneak a peek in the trolleys around you and notice that the ones filled with low-fat, no added sugar, reduced calorie meals are typically being steered by someone who is struggling with their weight, and yet when you notice the person with the figure of a broom handle, their trolley is full of 'normal' food... chicken, beef, crisps, vegetables, maybe some wine or beer, in other words real food, not processed meals with all the flavour, and goodness, stripped out.

I heard of a study involving a group of nearly two dozen children aged between 18 months and 3 years old. For a period of 28 days, they were given access to all foods, 24 hours a day, seven days a week. If you're a parent, you might already be cringing at how you think this turned out, but you're probably very wrong in your assumptions. In less than a week, nearly all of them were eating a perfectly balanced diet. They may have had some strange combinations, potatoes dipped in yoghurt with a side order of nuts perhaps, but nutritionally they were mostly getting it right, however strange. How? Was it because they'd read the latest medical journal, or been given a bespoke nutritional plan? No, they were just following their instinct, eating what they wanted, the amounts they wanted, when they wanted to.

If I ask you not to think of a blue tree, what the first thing you think about? A blue tree, right? So what do you think happens when you decide to eat healthy food, depriving yourself of the stuff you like? That's right, all your attention goes on the food you're trying to avoid because you spend a lot of the time thinking about it, tell yourself how good you've been not having donuts, or checking how long since your last candy bar. Remember what happens when you're waiting on delivery of your new car or baby? You would begin to find them everywhere, and this is no different, you would begin to find temptation and opportunity everywhere. So here's what I'm going to ask you to do…

Eat food you enjoy, not food you endure!

If I suggested you only eat foods that taste like old shoes with the texture to match, how likely would you to be to keep it up (assuming you don't enjoy eating old shoes)? Probably not very, so by giving yourself permission to eat the foods you enjoy, there is no forbidden fruit (sorry, couldn't resist) that you have to deny yourself. You'll also find that as you begin to accept that food is no longer the enemy, but simply a fuel, you'll begin to spend less time thinking about it, except when you're actually eating. As a result, you'll also begin to enjoy food more, but I'll talk about that later.

Every 7 to 14 days you develop a new set of tastebuds, this is one of the reasons to try new foods several times over a period of weeks. This gives you the chance to develop a taste for them, but it also means that the foods you enjoy and indeed crave can also change. It's also the reason that allowing children the opportunity to taste new foods several times over a period of time is more likely to encourage them to enjoy it, as it provides the opportunity for their taste to change, making the food more palatable.

We've all heard about women who experience cravings during pregnancy, some of which can be startlingly weird. I've personally heard from women who had cravings for coal, sponge (the kind you find at the bottom of the sea, not in the bakers), and weirdest of all, fire lighter blocks! Now, I'm not recommending any of these, but simply highlighting that the body knows what it needs, and will endeavour to meet the needs for proteins, vitamins, calcium or whatever it is it needs by creating a craving for certain foods. During pregnancy, it's the body's way of saying, "This is what I need to make another human being."

If you've ever felt a little less than ideal the morning after a small glass of what tickled your fancy, which I'm sure you probably only had for medicinal purposes, then you understand what a hangover feels like. At some point you may have declared, "I know what'll sort me out... _____" You can fill in your own blank here, but it's your body letting you know what it needs to repair the damage done the night before.

These are simply examples of your body sending signals to let you know what it is it wants, although in the case of pregnancy cravings, these should be tempered with a little common sense. It's simply that you had learned to tune out these signals, unless they got really demanding, but they are always there. As you are learning to spend less and less time obsessing with foods you're 'not allowed', you'll find you can become more aware of these signals that you are constantly sending yourself. You may even surprise yourself from time to time, and develop a taste for something you believed you didn't like, and yet thoroughly enjoy every mouthful when you do eat it.

You probably know someone who eats all the foods you considered "forbidden" whilst maintaining a healthy body. This clearly demonstrates that how you eat is as important as what you eat, not that what you eat doesn't play an important part, but it's not the only part!

As we've discussed how and when you eat affects your metabolism, and so does what you eat. The presence of certain nutrients can help speed up your metabolism leading to weight loss, and similarly, the absence of certain nutrients can slow your metabolism down, leading to weight gain.

In particular, certain food groups can speed up your metabolism:

- Proteins can increase your metabolic rate by up to 30%

- Carbohydrates can increase your metabolic rate up to 6%

- Fats can increase your metabolic rate up to 4%

Using the above information, starting your meals with protein can help to 'kick start' your metabolism to more efficiently process carbohydrates and fats.

People who have a weight problem can commonly have vitamin B deficiencies, in particular vitamin B12 which metabolise carbohydrates, so eating foods rich in B12 can be hugely beneficial in helping your body process carbohydrates properly. these foods include fish and shellfish, fortified cereals & soy products, red meat, low fat dairy products, cheese and eggs.

One of the key elements in successful weight loss is a varied and comprehensive diet. Mix it up, don't have the same foods all the time. Changing what you consume regularly keeps your metabolism active.

Chapter 8

Success Hacking

Solving the puzzle

If you simply carry on doing the same things, the same way you've always done them, you're going to keep getting the results you've always got. So by making small changes across all areas of your life you can stack the odds for success in your favour. Do you remember the Rubik's Cube? It's all very well understanding how all the parts move, but learning in which order you have to move them is the key to unlocking the solution.

By making small changes in your thinking, behaviours and routines, you will begin to find the ones that *really* work for you until you unlock the solution that propels you towards success.

There are lots of little changes you can make to create lasting change in your own behaviours around food and the relationship you have with it.

Tip 1: If you've ever gone shopping on an empty stomach, you know how much extra, impulse food you buy, because you were easily able to imagine how good it would be to eat it right there and then. So how do you stop pit happening? Always go shopping on a full stomach, and stick to your pre-planned shopping list, and only take the right amount of money with you.

Tip 2: Make sure you avoid 'ready meals' and go for the healthier option - that does NOT mean the 'diet' version, it means fresh fruit, vegetables and meat so you can prepare the meal yourself, knowing that every ingredient is promoting your new healthy life style. There are so many chemicals, preservatives, additives, sweeteners and more that are sometimes added to ready meals that it's hard to keep track which ones actually make the meal healthier, and which ones don't.

Tip 3: Plan meals and snacks in advance, carry snacks with you so that if you find yourself unexpectedly hungry, while away from home, you are still able to make choices about which foods you eat.

Tip 4: Don't keep food out on display on worktops or shelves, as this can give way to picking at foods unnecessarily, and only have healthy foods in the house, removing the temptation to eat 'junk' foods.

Tip 5: Consider the triggers that caused problems for you in the past, and plan how to avoid those 'stimulus'. This can be feelings, thoughts, events or situation. Find a way to remove these triggers, and develop a strategy for dealing with them when they happen unexpectedly. Practising relaxation techniques, limited exposure to help you build tolerance, or making a substitution that leads to a better outcome, can all help you to develop better behaviours that can be integrated at the unconscious level through repetition.

Pay attention to who or what is the triggers for you - even keep a diary to build up a bigger picture of what was happening to create the problems.

This can help you to identify:

- Timing of unwanted behaviour

- Events that happen prior to unwanted behaviour

- Place that the unwanted behaviour occurs

- With whom the unwanted behaviour occurs

- How you feel before and after the unwanted behaviour

If at some point you have a lapse, the important thing is that you identify what led to it happening, so that you can prevent it from recurring.

Tip 6: Have a small piece (about the size of an oxo cube) of protein before going to bed. This helps to prevent catabolism (the breaking down of complex molecules), which results in the body having less muscle and more fat. When eating this small amount of protein, it is broken down for the body processes, preventing catabolism happening. The best protein to have is cottage cheese, as it contains a slow release protein that keeps the body absorbing amino acids for several hours. Avoid fatty snacks such as chicken with the skin still on, or high fat meats including lamb or beef.

Tip 7: If you are microwaving food to reheat it, do *not* use plastic containers, as these release aluminium which slows down your metabolism.

Tip 8: Variety in your meal choices will keep your metabolism in shock, and therefore keep it working. Whilst it's easy to eat the same things day after day, it wont help your metabolism.

Chapter 9

Measurements

You know those mornings when everything is going great, you awaken feeling great and bounce out of bed when the alarm goes off, you catch yourself singing in the shower, you put on your favourite clothes, look in the mirror and feel *great*. Then you step on the scales and your world crumbles as you realise your weight has gone in the opposite direction from where you want. A moment ago you still weighed the same, and you were feeling great, and now it's a completely different story, not because your weight has suddenly changed, but because your *thinking* has changed in response to the experience you've just had. When you were measuring your success on how your clothes looked and felt on your body, you felt good! So if you *must* see a number changing, use measurements as everyones weight fluctuates, and measurements will give you a more consistent way to track your progress. Use the chart at the end of this chapter to record your measurements, following the instructions below.

How To Measure

When recording your own measurements, it's important you make sure you are measuring correctly to accurately track your success.

You don't need to use all the measurements, but the more measurements you track, the better the overall picture of your success you will build up.

Thighs: Let your hand fall by your side and measure around the thigh where you finger tip lands.

Hips: Place the measuring tape around at the widest part of the hips/buttocks keeping the tape parallel to the floor.

Waist: Place the measuring tape about 1/2 inch above the belly button (typically the narrowest part of the waist) and measure after you exhale, but before you inhale again.

Chest: Place the tape just under the bust/pecs keeping the tape parallel to the floor.

Bust: Place the tape across the nipples, measuring around the largest part of the chest with the tape parallel to the floor.

Biceps: Measure the largest part of the arm between the elbow and shoulder.

Neck: Measure around the largest part of the neck.

	Thighs	Hips	Waist	Chest	Bust	Biceps	Neck
Week 1							
Week 2							
Week 3							
Week 4							
Week 5							
Week 6							
Week 7							
Week 8							
Week 9							
Week 10							

Chapter 10

Stay Hydrated

Water, Water, Everywhere

You've probably, at one time or another, found yourself staring blankly in to the kitchen cupboard, asking yourself, "What do I want?" This is commonly a sign of dehydration, as you find that no matter what you have, it doesn't quite hit the mark! Sometimes it's the endorphin rush associated with "feel good" foods that you were craving, however by following the steps mentioned earlier regarding being more active, you will find those cravings happening less and less, as by being more active, you have endorphins rushing through your system more of the time, making you feel more happier and more content, more of the time.

Most people underestimate the importance of staying properly hydrated. Allowing your body to become dehydrated can result, in the short term, with people experiencing light headaches or dizziness, tiredness, and inability to concentrate fully. Long term it can lead to pressure ulcers, constipation and kidney or gallstones.

The reason it can also affect weight management is if your body becomes dehydrated, initially your body will prioritise your primary organs, and so will draw fluids from other parts of the body. When your primary organ function becomes affected, your kidneys can no longer filter your blood of impurities properly, and so your liver begins to take up some of the slack, reducing liver function which stops it from breaking down fats to produce energy, meaning the fat simply get stored.

As a guide, it's widely accepted that eight 8 ounce glasses of water per day is in the right ball park, or 2 litres over the course of a day. It's equally important that it's not all consumed in one sitting, as this can have an adverse affect of the body, so make sure you spread it out over the day. Remember this is only a guideline - personally, I have 2-3 litres of unflavoured sparkling water every day, sometimes more if I've had alcohol or caffeine.

Some people find carrying a water bottle with them helps to achieve the recommended amount. Remember that any drinks that do not have a diuretic effect also count towards this, so unsweetened fruit teas count towards the recommended amount. Caffeinated teas and coffees have a diuretic effect so if you do drink these, drink water afterwards to minimise the effect and to help flush the kidneys.

Make sure you note down *all* your drinks in the food diary, so you can identify which ones are promoting a healthy level of hydration, and which ones are detracting from maintaining your hydration levels, and then consider what adjustments you can make to your habits and routines to ensure you stay hydrated and don't mistake thirst for genuine hunger.

Conclusion

Everything You Need Is Already Within You

Hopefully now you realise you're far more like Dorothy with her red slippers, than an out of control roller coaster with no end in sight. No, there isn't a magic spell in this book, other than perhaps the one that helps you to wake up to your own personal power and your ability to take control of your future through the choices, decisions and actions that you take from this day forward.

Never before have we had access to such a breadth and depth of knowledge about how our minds and bodies work in a symbiotic relationship, and once we learn to use this to our advantage by resetting back to our natural defaults, a healthy mind *and* body are your for the taking.

By following the simple steps laid out in this book, you too can reset back to the best, healthiest version of yourself.

If I was to distill the essence of this book, it would be this...

- Eat when you are hungry

- Stop when you are full

- Eat Consciously

- Eat the food you enjoy

Sure, as we make our way through life some things require immense effort and superhuman skills, combined with unwavering determination. Being healthy isn't one of those things. Being healthy simply requires you to know how all the pieces work, and to pay attention to make sure you are moving forwards and not backwards. If you find yourself going back the way, it's only a problem if you don't choose to make a change.

Now it's over to you to start making better choices and decisions, and living a healthier life.

Resources

If you would like to join the Get Serious Get Slim community, then visit:

www.nlptransformations.org.uk/ getslim/

You will be given access to hypnosis downloads, weight management hints & tips, along with healthy, nutritious recipes.

Authors

Barry & Marina Collins are the husband and wife team that make up Transformations, dedicated to helping people find their way in the world, whether it's weight management or dealing stress & anxiety, the key to your unconscious is what makes them so effective at creating lasting change.

Although they will turn their attention where it's needed, their passion lies in helping individuals overcome fear. That sometimes comes in the form of spiders, flying, needles or balloons, but they will frequently use firewalking as a metaphor for the fears we *all* face in life, and feel held back by. Certified Firewalk instructors under The Firewalking Centre, the home of Tolly Burkan, they have taken hundreds of people safely across red hot coals, helping them break through fears and limiting beliefs in a matter of hours.

Find out more at:

www.nlptransformations.org.uk

www.phoenixfirewalk.uk

22985081R00054

Printed in Great Britain
by Amazon